Kegel Exercises Guide For Beginners

A Complete Kegel Exercise Guide Enhancing Strength Twice Gains And Bodybuilding Tips

Vicky Klocko

Table of Contents

CHAPTER ONE
Introduction

Kegel exercises involve contracting and relaxing the pelvic floor muscles. These exercises are designed to strengthen the pelvic floor, which supports the bladder, uterus, rectum, and other pelvic organs.

The pelvic floor muscles are crucial for various bodily functions such as controlling urination, bowel movements, and sexual function. Weakness in these muscles can lead to urinary incontinence, pelvic organ prolapse, and other issues.

Performing Kegel exercises regularly can help:

Improve bladder control: Strengthening these muscles can reduce instances of urinary incontinence or leakage, especially in women after childbirth or menopause.

Enhance sexual function: Strong pelvic floor muscles can contribute to improved sexual sensation and orgasmic response.

Prevent pelvic organ prolapse: Strengthening the pelvic floor can reduce the risk of pelvic organs sagging or slipping out of place.

Kegel exercises involve identifying the pelvic floor muscles, which are the ones you'd use to stop the flow of urine or prevent passing gas. Once identified, the exercises consist of contracting these muscles, holding the contraction for a few seconds, and then relaxing. It's important not to flex other muscles, like those in the abdomen, thighs, or buttocks, during these exercises.

To ensure effectiveness, it's recommended to do Kegel exercises regularly, starting with a few repetitions and gradually increasing the number as the muscles strengthen. Consulting a healthcare professional, particularly a pelvic floor physical therapist, can provide tailored guidance on performing Kegel exercises correctly.

Performing Kegel Exercises

Identifying and targeting the pelvic floor muscles is essential for effective Kegel exercises:

Identifying the Pelvic Floor Muscles:

Stop the Flow: To identify these muscles, try stopping the flow of urine while you're using the restroom. However, don't make a habit of regularly stopping urine flow as it can disrupt normal bladder emptying.

Squeeze and Lift: Another way to identify these muscles is by imagining you're trying to prevent passing gas. The muscles you use to do this are your pelvic floor muscles.

Proper Technique for Kegel Exercises: Once you've identified these muscles, follow these steps:

Get Comfortable: Sit, stand, or lie down in a comfortable position.

Empty Your Bladder: It's advisable to empty your bladder before starting Kegel exercises.

Contract the Muscles: Squeeze your pelvic floor muscles. Focus on the muscles you identified earlier, specifically the sensation of lifting and tightening them.

Hold the Contraction: Hold the squeeze for about 3-5 seconds, gradually working up to 10 seconds as you get stronger. Remember to breathe normally during this time.

Relax: Release the muscles and rest for the same amount of time as you held the contraction. This allows the muscles to recover.

Repeat: Aim for 10-15 repetitions in one session. Gradually increase this number as your muscles strengthen.

Tips for Effective Kegel Exercises

Consistency is Key: Perform Kegel exercises regularly, ideally multiple times a day.

Avoid Overdoing It: Don't overwork your pelvic floor muscles by doing too many repetitions at once. Gradually increase reps over time.

Stay Focused: Ensure you're isolating the pelvic floor muscles without tensing other muscles like the abdomen, thighs, or buttocks.

Breathing: Focus on maintaining regular breathing throughout the exercise.

Seek Guidance: If unsure about technique or if you're not seeing results, consider consulting a healthcare professional or a pelvic floor physical therapist for guidance.

Remember, like any exercise routine, it may take time to notice improvements. Consistency and proper technique are crucial for effectiveness.

Benefits of Kegel Exercises

Absolutely, Kegel exercises offer numerous benefits, particularly in terms of bladder control and overall pelvic health:

Improving Bladder Control:

Reducing Urinary Incontinence: Kegel exercises are known to significantly reduce urinary incontinence, especially in women post-pregnancy or during menopause.

Controlling Urges: Strengthening the pelvic floor muscles can help in better controlling sudden urges to urinate, reducing incidents of urgency incontinence.

Post-Surgery Recovery: For individuals who have undergone prostate surgery (in men) or pelvic surgery (in women), Kegel exercises can aid in quicker recovery of bladder control.

Enhancing Pelvic Health:

Preventing Pelvic Organ Prolapse: Strengthening the pelvic floor muscles provides support to pelvic organs, reducing the risk of pelvic organ prolapse, where organs like the bladder, uterus, or rectum can drop or bulge into the vagina.

Improved Sexual Function: Enhanced pelvic floor strength can lead to improved sexual sensations and more intense orgasms for both men and women.

Preventive Health Measures: Strengthening these muscles may prevent or alleviate discomfort associated with certain pelvic health issues, including constipation, fecal incontinence, and chronic pelvic pain.

CHAPTER TWO

Establishing a Kegel Routine

Incorporating Kegel exercises into your daily routine can be beneficial for consistency and effectiveness:

Set Reminders: Incorporate Kegel exercises into your daily schedule by setting reminders on your phone or associating them with a regular activity, like brushing your teeth or meal times.

Create a Plan: Decide on the number of repetitions and sets you aim to do each day. Start with a manageable amount and gradually increase as you get stronger.

Variety: Include Kegel exercises at different times during the day to ensure consistency. For example, do some in the morning, some during lunch, and others in the evening.

Track Progress: Keep a journal or use an app to track your exercises. Monitoring progress can motivate you to stick to your routine.

Tips for Consistency

Link to Habits: Pairing Kegel exercises with existing habits, like morning stretches or before bedtime rituals, can make it easier to remember.

Make it Enjoyable: If possible, make your routine enjoyable. Find a comfortable and relaxing environment to perform the exercises.

Be Patient: Results may take time. Don't get discouraged if you don't notice immediate improvements. Consistency is key.

Accountability: Consider involving a partner or friend in your routine for added motivation and accountability.

Reward System: Implement a reward system for yourself to celebrate milestones and consistency. It could be something as simple as treating yourself to something you enjoy after completing a week or a month of consistent exercises.

Advanced Kegel Techniques

Advancing in Kegel exercises involves gradually increasing the difficulty and exploring variations to further strengthen the pelvic floor muscles:

Gradual Progression and Challenges:

Extended Hold: Once you're comfortable with standard Kegel exercises, gradually increase the duration of each contraction. Start with holding for 5-10 seconds and work up to 10-20 seconds per contraction.

Increased Repetitions: Gradually increase the number of repetitions in each set. Aim to build up to 20-30 repetitions per session.

Quick Contractions: Introduce quick, rapid contractions of the pelvic floor muscles. Contract and relax the muscles rapidly for about 2-3 seconds each, repeating this in sets.

Add Resistance: Some devices or weights are available specifically designed to add resistance to Kegel exercises, providing an added challenge to strengthen the muscles.

Variations for Increased Strength

Elevated Positions: Try performing Kegels in different positions like standing or on your toes. These variations engage the muscles differently, enhancing their strength.

Combine with Exercise: Incorporate Kegel exercises into other exercises, such as squats or lunges, to engage the pelvic floor along with larger muscle groups.

Bridge Pose: Practice the yoga bridge pose, which engages the pelvic floor muscles along with the core and glutes.

Pilates and Yoga: Both Pilates and certain yoga poses emphasize core strength, which can indirectly strengthen the pelvic floor muscles.

Biofeedback Techniques: Some advanced techniques involve using biofeedback devices or apps that provide real-time feedback on muscle contractions. These can help ensure you're targeting and strengthening the correct muscles.

Always proceed gradually and listen to your body. If you experience any discomfort or pain, scale back and reassess your technique.

Pregnancy and Postpartum Benefits

Kegel exercises offer specific benefits for both pregnancy/postpartum health and men's health:

During Pregnancy: Strengthening the pelvic floor muscles can help prepare for childbirth by potentially reducing the risk of urinary incontinence during pregnancy and supporting the pelvic organs as the uterus grows.

Postpartum Recovery: After childbirth, practicing Kegel exercises can aid in the recovery of pelvic floor strength, potentially reducing urinary incontinence and supporting the healing process. However, it's crucial to consult with a healthcare professional for guidance on when to start and how to perform these exercises postpartum.

Benefits for Men's Health

Improved Bladder Control: Kegel exercises can benefit men by improving bladder control, particularly in cases of urinary incontinence after prostate surgery.

Erectile Dysfunction: Some studies suggest that Kegel exercises might help improve erectile dysfunction by enhancing blood circulation to the pelvic region and strengthening the pelvic floor muscles. However, their effectiveness might vary among individuals.

Prostate Health: Strengthening the pelvic floor muscles can support prostate health and potentially aid in preventing or managing issues related to prostate conditions.

For both these specific situations, it's essential to perform Kegel exercises correctly.

CHAPTER THREE

Maintaining Pelvic Health

Maintaining pelvic health involves more than just Kegel exercises; lifestyle factors play a significant role:

Healthy Weight: Maintaining a healthy weight can reduce the strain on the pelvic floor muscles and organs, supporting overall pelvic health.

Regular Exercise: Engaging in regular physical activity can strengthen the pelvic floor indirectly by supporting core muscles and promoting overall fitness.

Proper Posture: Maintaining good posture can alleviate unnecessary pressure on the pelvic floor and surrounding muscles.

Healthy Diet: A balanced diet rich in fiber can prevent constipation, which, if chronic, can strain the pelvic floor muscles.

Avoidance of Straining: Avoid activities that put excessive strain on the pelvic floor, such as heavy lifting or high-impact exercises without proper form.

Long-Term Benefits of Kegel Exercises

Sustained Bladder Control: Consistent practice of Kegel exercises can help maintain bladder control as one ages, reducing the risk of urinary incontinence.

Preventive Measures: Strengthening the pelvic floor muscles can act as a preventive measure against pelvic organ prolapse and other pelvic floor-related issues.

Enhanced Sexual Health: Maintaining strong pelvic floor muscles can contribute to improved sexual function and pleasure over time.

Overall Quality of Life: By supporting pelvic health, Kegel exercises can contribute to a better quality of life, allowing individuals to engage in daily activities without concerns about bladder control or pelvic discomfort.

Incorporating Kegel exercises into a healthy lifestyle regimen and performing them consistently over the long term can provide lasting benefits for pelvic health. However, it's important to strike a balance and ensure a holistic approach to overall health while considering the pelvic region's specific needs.

Embracing Kegel Exercises for Wellness

Embracing Kegel exercises as part of your wellness routine can bring about significant benefits for pelvic health and overall well-being. By focusing on these exercises, you're investing in a crucial aspect of your body that supports various functions and contributes to your quality of life.

Kegel exercises offer a multitude of advantages, from improving bladder control and enhancing sexual function to preventing pelvic organ prolapse and supporting postpartum recovery. Incorporating these exercises into your daily routine, along with maintaining a healthy lifestyle, can amplify their long-term benefits.

Remember, consistency is key. Starting gradually, identifying the pelvic floor muscles, and gradually increasing the difficulty over time can ensure effectiveness and sustainability. Additionally, seeking guidance from healthcare professionals, especially pelvic floor physical therapists, can provide personalized insights and ensure you're performing these exercises correctly.

Ultimately, embracing Kegel exercises as part of your wellness journey empowers you to take proactive steps toward maintaining pelvic health and enjoying a better quality of life. By making them a regular part of your routine, you're prioritizing your well-being and nurturing an essential aspect of your body's health.

Conclusion

Kegel exercises offer a simple yet powerful way to strengthen the pelvic floor muscles, supporting bladder control, sexual function, and overall pelvic health. These exercises involve identifying and contracting the pelvic floor muscles, with benefits ranging from reducing urinary incontinence to enhancing postpartum recovery and improving men's health.

Understanding the importance of pelvic floor health and incorporating Kegel exercises into your daily routine can pave the way for long-term benefits. Consistency, proper technique, gradual progression, and considering lifestyle factors contribute to maximizing the effectiveness of these exercises.

By embracing Kegel exercises as part of your wellness regimen, you're not only nurturing your pelvic health but also investing in a better quality of life.

floor muscles, supporting bladder control, sexual function, and overall pelvic health. These exercises involve identifying and contracting the pelvic floor muscles, with benefits ranging from reducing urinary incontinence to enhancing postpartum recovery and improving men's health.

Understanding the importance of pelvic floor health and incorporating Kegel exercises into your daily routine can pave the way for long-term benefits. Consistency, proper technique, gradual progression, and considering lifestyle factors contribute to maximizing the effectiveness of these exercises.

By embracing Kegel exercises as part of your wellness regimen, you're not only nurturing your pelvic health but also investing in a better quality of life.

THE END